The Ultimate Fibromyalgia Book Guide

How to Successfully Live with Fibromyalgia and Recipes for the Fibromyalgia Diet

Mia Soleil

Table of Contents

Introduction

I want to thank you and congratulate you for purchasing this book.

This book contains treatments, strategies and recipes on how to successfully live with fibromyalgia and manage your pain.

Fibromyalgia is a chronic condition that influences more than 5 million people, a large majority being women. The constant pain and fatigue from fibromyalgia robs the individual from enjoying everyday life. Trying to find ways to manage and cope with this disorder can be very taxing to those who are affected by it.

I, too, have suffered from chronic pain and have felt its daily debilitating effects. I know the frustration of living a life packed with medical appointments, aggravation, discouragement and hopelessness. Fibromyalgia can be ruthless, unrelenting and difficult to conquer however things can turn around for the better.

My desire for you is to find encouragement and relief from your fibromyalgia through this book. I hope you will find treatments and lifestyle adjustments that you can make in your everyday life to help rein in this beast. Take heart, there is hope. Be strong. Preserve, pursue and fight for a life at peace with fibromyalgia.

I wish you luck on your path to wellness. To help you achieve the better version of yourself, I and my colleagues at Joy Publishing invite you to like our Facebook Page: www.facebook.com/joypublishing. Get free books and know of our new releases by joining us.

I sincerely thank you again for purchasing this book. I truly hope you enjoy it! Please take some time to stop by and LIKE our Facebook page:

https://www.facebook.com/joypublishing

With gratitude,

Mia Soleil

Chapter 1 - Dealing with Fibromyalgia

Fibromyalgia is classified as a non-threatening, chronic disorder. It is associated with a widespread pain in the musculoskeletal system accompanied with mood, stress, fatigue and sleep issues. It must be understood that fibromyalgia is not considered a disease, but a syndrome. It won't threaten your life, but the pain may become unbearable at any given time.

Most sufferers describe the condition as having persistent flu-like symptoms with pain being felt all over the body. The pain that it causes can be so severe that it has been linked to many cases of anxiety, headaches and even depression.

Although there is no scientific proof yet that having a proper diet and doing healthy lifestyle changes can indeed alleviate the symptoms of fibromyalgia, sufferers of the condition who chose to do modifications to their lifestyle and diet have seen significant improvement. If it worked for them, it will certainly do anyone suffering from the condition some good too, including you.

The Pain Is Not Just in Your Head

Because fibromyalgia is practically invisible, meaning x-rays or most lab tests do not and cannot give measurable findings regarding the condition, it does not mean that the pain you feel is just in your head. The pain is indeed real. The pain may not have any ability to inflict damage on the organs of your body or your joints but the relentless experience of being in pain can leave a significant influence in dealing with daily life.

The pain that comes with fibromyalgia can be so intense but without medical tests that can confirm it some sufferers are convinced that the pain they feel is only in their heads and that there is really no actual body pain. They think that their brain is just playing a nasty trick on them.

Currently, the medical community acknowledges the fact that the pain that is associated with having fibromyalgia is real. According to a research, it may be caused by a glitch in the manner that the body perceives or senses the pain. The researchers believe that the condition intensifies the pain sensation by influencing the processing of pain signals in the brain.

The symptoms sometimes start after a major psychological stress, surgery, physical trauma or infection. There are also cases where symptoms slowly progress within a certain period of time with an unknown trigger.

Risk Factors and Complications

Women are more likely to have fibromyalgia than men and it is also possible to develop it if someone in your family has the condition too. Individuals with lupus or rheumatoid arthritis and other rheumatic diseases are also more likely to have fibromyalgia.

Several individuals who have fibromyalgia also experience having temporomandibular joint (TMJ) disorders, tension headaches, depression, anxiety and irritable bowel syndrome (IBS).

Fibromyalgia can also lead to other problems and may make life even more difficult. The pain and lack of good sleep due to fibromyalgia can no doubt impede your ability to function properly at work or at home. The frustrations of handling the often misunderstood condition can lead to health-related anxiety and depression.

Today, there is still no known cure for fibromyalgia, but there are available medications that can help alleviate the symptoms and let you go through the day without so much trouble. Good diet, exercise, stress-reduction procedures, rest and relaxation may also help in improving the symptoms of this condition.

It is best to take necessary measures and start practicing a healthy lifestyle if you are someone who is at risk in developing the condition or has the condition already. Eating a well-balanced diet, avoiding certain foods, having a regular workout routine and maintaining a stress-free life can help a lot in keeping your condition under control.

Symptoms of Fibromyalgia

The most typical symptom of fibromyalgia is a widespread pain (the sufferer experiences pain on both sides of the body, as well as above and below the waist) which usually lasts for at least three months. There are cases wherein pain literally becomes a typical occurrence in the daily life of the victim. The pain can disturb the day to day existence of its victims especially those with a low pain threshold.

Sufferers of fibromyalgia often wake up in the morning feeling sluggish and tired even though they slept for many hours during the night. Their sleep is often interrupted by pain; in fact, several fibromyalgia victims also have sleep disorders like sleep apnea and restless legs syndrome.

Many individuals who suffer from fibromyalgia may also have constant headaches and cramps in the lower abdomen. There also exists a symptom that is typically referred to as "fibro fog" which impairs the ability of those with fibromyalgia to focus and concentrate on the work at hand.

Possible Causes of Fibromyalgia

Medical experts are still baffled regarding the real culprits or causes of fibromyalgia, but it is suspected that several factors that come together make the pain as intense as it is.

It is suspected that fibromyalgia may be an inherited condition. Scientific studies have been investigating genetic mutations or genetic markers that may be present in those who have fibromyalgia and their families.

There are also other conditions that may trigger the occurrence of fibromyalgia or make it much worse. Some experts believe that post-traumatic stress disorder (PTSD) can be one of the triggers the disease.

Women and Fibromyalgia

Around 80% to 90% of people diagnosed with fibromyalgia are women. The reason for such number may have something to do with the genes, hormones and differences in the immune system between the two sexes. Still, researchers are not exactly sure why women have the greater number of fibromyalgia sufferers than men.

Women who suffer from fibromyalgia often describe their pain as a dull ache that begins in the muscles. Sufferers experience pain on both sides of the body which also affects the upper and lower body parts. The pain can usually come and go for a period of at least three months. In some days, the pain can be so severe that it makes it impossible for a woman to stick with the planned activities for the day.

Many women with fibromyalgia have trouble keeping their focus and remembering things. They often mix up words when they talk or get confused more quickly than normal. These problems are collectively referred to as "fibro fog" because their minds feel foggy. Medical researchers are not quite certain regarding the cause of fibro fog, but they suspect that the lack of sleep or the effects on the brain of fibromyalgial pain may be the ones causing it.

Moreover, around half of fibromyalgia sufferers develop headaches. Several women get a throbbing headache or a migraine which can cause vomiting and nausea. The reasons for such an occurrence of headaches in fibromyalgia patients are still a mystery. Experts believe that the imbalance of chemicals in the brain, such as epinephrine and serotonin, may be the cause of the recurrent headaches.

One bodily system greatly affected in women with fibromyalgia is the reproductive system. One common symptom present in patients with fibromyalgia is menstrual cramps. These menstrual cramps can be extremely painful or just mild. Not all women experience these camps, but most women with fibromyalgia have more painful menstrual periods than normal. Some women with fibromyalgia also develop endometriosis in which the tissue from the uterus extends in some parts of the pelvis. Another problem that females with fibromyalgia experience is dyspareunia or painful sexual intercourse.

The digestive system is also affected by fibromyalgia. Irritable bowel syndrome or IBS is common in women who have fibromyalgia. IBS is characterized by symptoms like bloating, diarrhea, constipation and stomach cramps. Researchers are yet to discover the real reason behind the connection between IBS and fibromyalgia.

Sensitivity is another issue that most women with fibromyalgia must face. Most women who developed such sensitivity may find themselves grabbing their sweater whenever the temperature drops or experience profuse sweating when the temperature suddenly shoots up. Some women with fibromyalgia are also sensitive to bright lights and/or loud noises.

Tender Points

Aside from the widespread pain, fibromyalgia also creates tender points all over the body. These points are about as small as pennies and are called as such because they hurt when someone presses on them. You may feel the pain in some or all of the identified tender points.

These are all the possible tender points in the body:

- above the nape

- front portion of the neck

- area between the shoulders

- top portion of the chest (specifically, on the second rib)

- elbows

- upper portion of the buttocks

- hips

- insides of both knees

If you are in a lot of pain, it is possible that you have developedfibromyalgia. Although the evidence and facts regarding this dreadful condition can send shivers to the bones, it is still reassuring to know that it is not life-threatening. It could hinder you from giving out your best, but there are ways to alleviate the symptoms and still finish the task at hand without so much trouble. Make sure you seek professional help if you are suspicious of having fibromyalgia. This simple test using tender points is not a complete diagnosis and doctors can do much more to know and identify what disorder you are having.

Chapter 2 - Treatments and Other Ways to Stop Fibromyalgia from Ruining Your Life

Fibromyalgia sufferers can make the symptoms go away or at least lessen the severity of the symptoms with nutritious food, lifestyle changes and exercise. Studies reveal that enhanced physical fitness and having a certain diet can help alleviate the symptoms of fibromyalgia.

Therapy, acupuncture, counseling, pain medications and massage are also some of the things that may help sufferers in making the condition less debilitating.

Tests and Diagnosis for Fibromyalgia

Today, physicians can diagnose that a person is suffering from fibromyalgia based on where the pain is felt and how long it has been going on.

There is no laboratory test that can prove that a person has the condition, but through many diagnostic tests the doctor can rule out other possible conditions that have the same symptoms as fibromyalgia. The tests may involve, but not limited to, thyroid function tests, x-rays and blood tests.

Preparing for a Doctor's Appointment

Due to the several similarities of fibromyalgia with other conditions, the patient may need to see not just one doctor. The patient's family doctor may recommend or refer the patient to doctors with different specializations since the pain is felt in many parts of the body and may involve different bodily systems.

It is best to prepare a detailed journal of the symptoms, the list of foods taken, habits, work, usual sleep patterns or if there's some trouble sleeping. Changes observed in the present and a detailed medical history can help a lot in the early diagnosis of fibromyalgia. The patient also needs to prepare his family medical history, as well as medications and supplements that he has taken or is currently taking. It is also best that the patient prepare a list questions or clarifications that the he wants to ask the doctor before the actual visit.

Common Treatments and Medications

Not all treatments and medications may work for all fibromyalgia victims, but a healthy diet and exercise can improve the condition of anyone.

There are patients who rely on pain relievers such as acetaminophen, naproxen sodium or ibuprofen to alleviate the pain. Some doctors may even give a prescription pain reliever for severe cases. However, taking narcotics is not a wise move to make because it can lead to dependence on the said drugs and may also cause worsening of the pain.

Antidepressants may be prescribed to help ease the fatigue and pain associated with fibromyalgia and also to aid the patients in getting restful sleep.

Anti-seizure medications, commonly used to treat epilepsy, may also be prescribed to help reduce some of the pain. Gabapentin and pregabalin are two popular anti-seizure drugs that can help reduce the symptoms of fibromyalgia in some patients.

Therapy and Alternative Medicine

Therapy and alternative medicine may work with some fibromyalgia patients. Some individuals attest that their condition improved when they tried a certain therapy or alternative medicine although these claims lack scientific evidence and still need further study.

One of the oldest methods that health care providers still practice today is massage therapy. This therapy involves using different techniques in manipulating the muscles and soft tissues of the body. Massage can definitely relax the muscles, bring down the heart rate and relax the nerves. It can also enhance the joints' range of motion, as well as increase the production of the natural painkillers of the body. It can effectively relieve anxiety and stress if done properly.

One type of massage, craniosacral therapy or CST, is a massage therapy which targets specific pressure points on the head and neck. Researchers discovered that those who had craniosacral massage therapy reported experiencing less pain and anxiety after a few sessions. Traces of depression had also diminished and they saw significant improvements in doing daily activities.

Another method called Cognitive Behavioral Therapy or CBT may also help fibromyalgia patients. CBT helps fibromyalgia patients identify negative thought patterns and turn them into something useful or beneficial to them. Researchers in Spain who evaluated fibromyalgia sufferers who went through the said therapy and some with combined hypnosis found out that the patients improved and that their symptoms were relieved faster as compared to using medications or drugs for their treatment.

Acupuncture, an ancient practice that originated in China, is also used by some to help alleviate the symptoms of fibromyalgia. It aims to restore the normal balance of life forces through the use of fine needles. These fine needles are inserted through the skin in varying depths. Western theories believe that the needles in acupuncture are responsible for changing the flow of blood and the neurotransmitter levels in the spinal cord and in the brain. The science behind how it works is not fully understood. The question of if it does indeed work has not been verified either.

Other forms of therapy like yoga and tai chi may also help control the symptoms of fibromyalgia. The practices combine slow movements, meditation, relaxation, and deep breathing.

These treatments may help alleviate the symptoms of fibromyalgia, but the relief they provide may only be temporary. Some drugs may even inflict more harm to the body in the long run especially if they are not monitored by health providers. Lifestyle changes, dietary modification and exercise may still prove to be the most effective solutions in battling its symptoms.

Chapter 3 - Lifestyle Change for Fibromyalgia Sufferers

In order to win against fibromyalgia, it is necessary to make some lifestyle adjustments that will help the sufferer in easing the pain, if not making all of it go away.

Eat Healthy Foods

Eating a well balanced diet can help a lot in alleviating the symptoms of fibromyalgia. It is a known fact that the body has the ability to heal itself by providing it with all the right nutrients and vitamins that the cells need in order to fight off harmful diseases or conditions.

Find Ways to Reduce Stress

Finding some means to reduce stress may seem next to impossible especially if there is constant pain, but there are ways to minimize or even eliminate stress in your life. Careful planning is the key in reducing stress. Work out a plan that will limit emotional stress and overexertion by setting a time each day to enjoy utmost relaxation.

Completely changing daily routines to get some much needed relaxation is necessary. Stressful activities may be removed or lessened in order to give more time for a little bit of R&R. Make your daily activities predictable but enjoyable to lessen the stress.

If you know what will happen next, you will feel less distraught since you know what to expect. Stress management techniques such as meditation, deep breathing and getting massages may also help in relieving stress.

Adequate Sleep Is Important

Fatigue is one of the symptoms of fibromyalgia, that's why getting adequate sleep is fundamental in keeping all the symptoms at bay. Aside from setting ample sleeping time, practicing good sleeping habits like going to bed at the same time each night and waking up at the same time each morning can help a lot. It is also best to limit daytime naps to get sounder sleep at night. Watching TV or working on the computer should be discontinued at least 2 hours before going to sleep.

Keep A Regular Exercise Schedule

During the first few times, exercise may add to the bodily pain but doing the routine on a regular basis may soon decrease the symptoms of fibromyalgia. Exercises may include walking, biking and swimming. A physical therapist can also help the patient develop a simple exercise program at home.

Learn Pacing

It is equally important to keep activities on equal levels each day. Patients with fibromyalgia must be warned that doing too much on "good" days (where pain seems to be completely out of the picture) may yield more "bad" days in the future. A fibromyalgia sufferer must keep everything in moderation - meaning avoid overdoing things during the days when pain is less and almost doing nothing during the bad days when symptoms are at their worst.

Keep everything balanced by doing the work in exactly the same pace in all of the days regardless if a particular day is good or not. Again, do your best to keep all of your activities within schedule and establish a daily routine regardless of how you're feeling.

Maintaining a healthy lifestyle is not only good for fibromyalgia relief, but the overall health as well. People with fibromyalgia will be able to do away with drugs and other medications in the long run just by keeping a healthy lifestyle.

Chapter 4 - Exercises That Can Help Alleviate the Symptoms of Fibromyalgia

There are different exercises that can help ease the symptoms of fibromyalgia and make life easier for the sufferers. Many doctors suggest implementing a fitness or exercise program before considering any kind of medications or drugs. Even if the doctor prescribes a certain drug for the condition, staying active can play a huge role in making the pain go away.

How Much Exercise?

Some research show that having a workout for at least two times a week with a minimum of 25 minutes per session can yield significant improvement of the symptoms. It is prudent to start off with a low-to-moderate set of exercises like walking, water aerobics, swimming, biking, tai chi or yoga. Start slow then gradually increase the time and intensity of the exercise to a point that is still tolerable. Individuals with fibromyalgia must remember that it is imperative that they do not to overexert.

Warm up before working out. Gentle joint rotations can be done before exercise. Start from the toes and go all the way up to the neck. Do slow circular motions in clockwise and counter-clockwise until all the joints in the body can move smoothly. Bear in mind to keep everything in moderation and never take the rotations to the point where it can be painful.

Walk the Pain Away

Most health authorities list walking as the topmost form of exercise that can help ease the pain brought about by fibromyalgia. It is because walking is considered a low-impact exercise that is safe and easy to do. It improves blood circulation and can help bring oxygen to the muscles and decrease the stiffness as well as the pain.

Start by walking 10 minutes per day then gradually increase the duration to 30 minutes per day. It is best to walk every day at your most convenient time.

Warm Water Workout Can Be Good Too

Light exercise and warm water is a combination that can help soothe the pain away. According to research, women who do aquatic exercises in a heated pool for at least an hour thrice a week show fewer symptoms of fibromyalgia than those who did not do the workout.

Someone who would like to try the workout can start with ten minutes of warm up by walking in the water, followed by ten minutes of moderate water aerobics, twenty minutes of strength exercises then lastly, cooling down.

Stretch your Way to a Pain Free Life

Simple stretching, good posture and relaxation exercises can lessen the amount of pain. Take note that it is best to stretch the stiff muscles before and after completing a light aerobic exercise to avoid possible injury.

Stretch gently and make sure to never stretch to the point where it becomes painful. Hold the light stretches for 30 seconds. Daily stretching can provide a kind of lubrication to the joints and can send oxygen and nutrients to the muscles.

When stretching the calves, face the wall and place your hands flat against it (as if pushing the wall). Position your feet flat on the floor, with one foot in front of the other. Lean forward and feel the pull in your calves and Achilles tendons. Hold the position for thirty seconds and repeat the entire exercise two more times. Switch the position of the legs and repeat.

Lightly Lift

Strength training can also reduce the pain of fibromyalgia while improving the wellbeing of a person. Using resistance machines or lifting weights can benefit fibromyalgia patients a lot as long as the intensity is appropriate for the patient, it should be increased gradually and weights must be kept light.

Start at one to three pounds then slowly increase the weight and keep it under a manageable point; again, avoid overexertion.

Count in the Chores

If working out in a gym doesn't seem to give the expected benefits, then doing some chores in the house can also be considered as exercise for individuals with fibromyalgia. Activities like scrubbing and vacuuming can help ease the pain and improve bodily movement and function.

Doing at least thirty minutes of chores each day can help lessen the pain that fibromyalgia brings.

Isometrics

Sometimes regular strength training is painful, but an isometric chest press is another way to tone and strengthen your muscles. Isometric exercises involve tensing the muscles without stretching or moving the muscles.

Do the chest press by putting your arms at chest level then pressing your palms together as hard as you can. Hold the position for five seconds, and then take a five-second rest before repeating the whole cycle for at least four more times. Slowly build the time of holding the press up to 15 seconds (if not painful). Stop if the exercise brings in more pain.

There is no perfect exercise regimen for fibromyalgia patients. It is all a matter of trying many things out and finding what is best for you. When you discover the set of exercises that work for you, stick with it and make sure to do it regularly. For better guidance, you can also work with a physical therapist to come up with a personalized exercise routine.

Chapter 5 – Sugar: The Sweet Poison at the Root of It All

Glucose, fructose, sucrose, dextrose, lactose, brown rice syrup, corn syrup and cane juice: what do all of these have in common as well as 250 other chemical compounds? Sugar!! They are all examples of sugar - the sweet, delicious and natural substance commonly found in fruits, vegetables, dairy and grains. Sugar falls under the carbohydrate category of the food guide and is necessary in our body. Carbohydrates are the body's main source of energy which fuel all of our muscles and also our brain.

So how can something so delectable and natural be a problem? It might seem as though sugar is safe and good for the body since it comes from natural sources; but scientists have gathered proof that this sweet poison, contrary to popular belief, causes havoc in all of our cells when taken in excess. It is vital to look at the effects of sugar to the body in order to better understand how to conquer fibromyalgia.

According to Dr. Jacob Teitelbaum, MD from the Dr. Oz Show, an overgrowth of yeast or Candida is an underlying contributor to the incidence of fibromyalgia and other chronic conditions. Therefore, the solution is to rid the excessive growth of yeast from the body. However, just removing the excessive yeast is not enough because there will **always be a certain amount left in the body.** It is important to achieve a healthy balance of yeast in the digestive tract. To control the amount of yeast growth in the body, detoxing from sugar must be done since the primary food source of yeast is sugar.

The Problem with Too Much Sugar...

Sugar poses as a risk to our body and weakens our organs and immune system. It is estimated that sugar is around eight times more addictive than cocaine. It is a biological addiction, a disorder of the hormones and an error in the chemical balance in your body that causes cravings for sugars and other carbohydrates. Aside from the fact that sugar is the food source of yeast, sugar provides no nutritional benefits. Sugar is void of fiber, protein, minerals and enzymes. When you consume too much sugar, consequently, your body needs to make up for the lack of nutrients by borrowing these necessary nutrients, e.g. sodium, potassium, calcium and magnesium, from other parts of the body. You can imagine the long term effects on the body when it's trying to metabolize the constantly high amounts of sugar in it.

Probably the most dangerous thing about sugar is that it is in everything! Surprisingly, a can of tomato soup contains 4 teaspoons of sugar. You can find sugar hidden in peanut butter, tomato sauce, crackers, and many, many other products that would never seem to have a natural connection with sugar. Overconsumption fosters an acidic imbalance in our predominately alkaline body, which is another reason why sugar is a problem. I will go into further detail about alkalinity and acidity in the next chapter since understanding the pH balance in our body is crucial in order to combat fibromyalgia.

How Do You Know You're Addicted to Sugar?

A sugar addiction is connected with a persistent imbalance of blood sugar in the body. Below are observed behavioral and physiological symptoms of a sugar addiction:

- You have a craving for bread products, sugary beverages or sweets.

- You experience what is called a "food coma". It is the feeling of drowsiness and fatigue after a heavy meal when the body is trying to deal with the sugar influx.

- When you miss a meal, you get a feeling of lightheadedness. If your body is used to a high-energy, high-calorie intake during every meal, missing a meal can make your body go into withdrawal.

- After you eat something sweet, your body craves for more. This is due to the fructose in the sugar, which encourages the production of ghrelin, a substance that increases the feeling of hunger.

- You have become dependent on caffeine to get your body started. You keep looking for coffee and sodas in order to stay awake and keep going.

- You have a harder time losing weight compared to average people. This is not because of your genes and definitely not from being too fat. This is because your body is too busy dealing with all that sugar to actually start burning fat. Furthermore, the acidic environment created in your body makes it even harder to shed those pounds.

Usually, these can be alleviated or even completely removed by balancing your blood sugar. Here are the tried and tested methods to do just that:

- Eat more proteins. Protein promotes muscle-building and helps metabolize your excess fats.

- Eliminate sugar and empty carbohydrates from your diet. Eating healthy meals regularly should be sufficient for your energy needs.

- Eat more good fats, complex carbohydrates, fiber and essential nutrients. A craving for sugar can come from your body not getting enough nutrients. Fiber-rich foods are also great for detoxifying your body not only from the build-up of sugar, but also from fats and other toxins.

It is reported that sugar addiction is worse than other kinds of addiction. You might find that it is more difficult to win over your addiction since sugar is in almost everything you eat and drink. However, once you have decided to rid yourself of it, you'll see results that you will be proud of.

Now What??

There are a few options for treating the overgrowth of yeast and sugar in your body. A huge part of the equation is making a dietary lifestyle change. Some medical experts recommend Diflucan, an anti-fungal medication. You can consult your doctor about your condition and request for a prescription.

There are several books on Candida cleanses in the market that you can find. You could try " *Yeast Infection Guide: A Natural Candida Cure to Boost Your Immune System and Achieve*

Optimal Health with a Complete Candida Cleanse and Candida Diet" by Lily Phillips.

Another absolute essential is having a sugar detox. For guidance, try the book " *21 Day Sugar Detox Guide for Beginners: Lose Weight Quickly, Achieve Optimal Health, Feel Energized and Eliminate Sugar Cravings Naturally"* by Emma Rose.

Consuming probiotics such as acidophilus will help maintain a healthy digestive environment. Acidophilus can be found in dairy products, particularly yogurt. Acidophilus supplements are also available at local pharmacies. Another exceptional product is consuming kefir, which is cow's milk fermented in specific bacteria resulting in a sour-tasting drink. This product can be found in health food stores.

Chapter 6 - Alkaline or Acidic?

In its basic sense, the alkaline diet (also known as the acid ash diet, alkaline ash diet and alkaline acid diet) is based on the theory that certain foods have a significant effect on the pH of our body fluids such as blood, saliva and urine.

When our body is in an alkaline state, it functions the way it was intended to. Almost all of the food products that we consume, once digested and metabolized, release either an alkaline base or an acid base into our blood. Grains, meat, shellfish, milk, poultry, cheese and salt all produce acid, hence unbalancing the proper pH of our blood (which is slightly alkaline). This kind of diet, if continued and not counteracted by alkaline foods, can cause some serious side effects.

There are at least 10 benefits to bringing your body into an alkaline state:

1. *Improves energy levels*

2. *Improves immune function*

3. *Slows aging*

4. *Reduces pain and inflammation*

5. *Decreases weight*

6. *Promotes teeth and gum health*

7. *Neutralizes acid imbalance*

8. *Eliminates risk factors for certain diseases*

9. *Improves overall heart condition*

10. *Removes harmful toxins*

After regulating their body's pH and eliminating foods that cause an influx of acid in the body, some people have reported a decrease in fibromyalgia symptoms. If the body's pH level falls below 7 or above 7.45, severe health conditions can occur with death being the worst outcome. When the pH falls below or above what is normal, the body constantly balances and fine tunes in order to keep this delicate balance. As a result, it will take nutrients from other areas of the body (such as the bones) and do whatever it needs to do to maintain its alkaline state. Consider it this way: when garbage is left out on the street, the rats come. In the same way, when our body is in an acidic state, our immunity is compromised. Wherever **garbage is, diseases, cancers and** abnormalities are sure to follow.

Let us take this information into consideration. The fastest way to heal fibromyalgia is to bring the body into an alkaline state. This is profound information and is not often talked about in media. Society has indeed a lot of learning to do. If you want to know more about the alkaline diet, you can try " *Alkaline Diet Guide: Lose Weight Quickly, Achieve Optimal Health and Feel Energized with the Alkaline Diet and Alkaline Recipes*" by Emma Rose.

Chapter 7 – The Power of Hydration

The natural healing power of hydration may not be a familiar natural treatment for fibromyalgia but it is by far more essential than any other treatment presented in this book. The topic of water is so foundational, so crucial, so revolutionary, that it deserves to have a chapter of its own. It is of utmost importance for people to be educated about the water they are consuming on a daily basis to nourish their bodies.

Our body's biology is composed of 75% water. Therefore, it is imperative to keep the body hydrated in order for all the cells, muscles and organs to function at their optimal levels. Surprisingly, not all water is created the same. **Regardless of where you source your water, its basic chemical composition remains the same, H_2O.** However, the structure of water is not created equal. **Sometimes, your tap water may actually not be the best source water to consume.** Globally, bottled watered is considered a popular alternative to tap water. In some countries, it is unsafe to consume the tap water because it is **polluted with a variety of contaminants.** When considering our water source, there are some important factors to consider such as its oxidation rating and its pH level.

First of all, it's important to note that plastic water bottles are one of the world's top pollutants. Only 1 out of 6 plastic bottles are actually recycled. This poses huge implications on the environment on many different levels. While this does not directly impact fibromyalgia, the long term repercussions can pose a lot of damage to our health and environment.

That being said, the plastic bottles that bottled water come in leech harmful chemicals into the contained water that contribute to raising estrogen levels in the human body. Due to the long process that involves production, packaging and transportation, the bottled water resides in its plastic bottle for lengthy periods of time. Therefore, the plastic chemicals have a longer window of time to leak into our water source. These are chemicals that should not be introduced into our body since they wreak havoc and create long term health implications.

Furthermore, bottled water and tap water in some areas have a higher positive oxidation rating which is correlated to an increase in free radicals in the body. These water sources are contributing to the problem of diseases and cancers rather than helping prevent them. It's horrifying to discover that the tap water in my city, which is considered top quality, is actually worse than the 7-Up soda in relation to its oxidation rating. 7-Up rated at least +400 while the tap water in my area rated over +600! Bottled water has almost the same oxidation rating as 7-Up and power drinks.

Besides the oxidation rating factor, it is also essential to take into account the pH level of the water we consume. The pH level in our water source is incredibly important, especially when we are looking at ways to heal fibromyalgia. Bottled water falls below neutral with 5/6 acidity. An acidic pH level is not good considering that our body is alkaline. Tap water's pH level will depend on where you live. In my area, where water is top quality, tap water is neutral at 7 on the pH scale. In some areas, the water is neutralized to reduce rusting of the water pipes (isn't that nice?).

In addition, chlorine is added to remove bacteria from the water since water poisoning is one of the top causes of death in the world. In the summer, the city increases the chlorine level to accommodate for the hotter climate. Consequently, the chlorine in the water is instantly absorbed into the body which may cause problems with our liver.

The beauty of alkaline water is that is supports the alkaline balance in our body. Unfortunately, only 1% of the world is educated about the positive, life changing effects of alkaline water. Achieving an alkaline state can quickly be achieved by drinking alkaline water. You can also partner alkaline water with a diet rich in alkaline foods – which should basically consist of food taken from plant sources like fruits and vegetables. Consuming alkaline water is greatly beneficial to our health. Its pH should be around 8.5-9.5. It hydrates the body more efficiently than bottled or tap water and it also detoxifies the body by neutralizing the acids and removing harmful toxins.

One of the best sources of alkaline water on the market right now is Kangen water. Kangen water uses a filter system that is attached to your sink in order to filter the water and create an alkaline pH level. In addition, the system ionizes the tap water through electrolysis which produces a negative oxidation rating. That means it becomes an antioxidant and takes away the harmful free radicals from the body. Furthermore, Kangen water can be used for cooking and cleaning. It's shocking to see all the pesticides and chemicals that wash off your vegetables after you use Kangen water to clean them.

When you get your hands on Kangen water, try a full body water transfusion. Drink 1 ounce for every pound of body weight a day. For an average 140 lb woman, that's about a gallon a day! Drink the same amount for 21 days and watch your body heal itself from the inside out. It's incredible!

Chapter 8 - Recommended Fibromyalgia Diet: Foods to Eat and to Avoid

Some foods can make fibromyalgia worse than before and there are also foods that can help ease the pain. Knowing which foods to avoid and to eat can bring great improvements on the symptoms of fibromyalgia.

Foods to Eat

Eating the right amounts of fruits, vegetables, fats, seeds, legumes, grains, lean meats, and fats can bring significant improvement in your overall health and fitness.

If you are committed to creating an alkaline environment in your body, consuming alkalizing foods will help you get there. Pretty much all fruits and vegetables are alkalizing – especially the green ones like wheat grass, kale, spinach, etc.

Try these excellent food choices:

- rich in fiber - green leafy vegetables, bran (particularly corn; also wheat, rice and oat), raw cauliflower, broccoli, cabbage, berries (particularly raspberries), celery, squash, beans (especially kidney beans), cooked white mushrooms, oranges, figs, nuts and seeds

- omega 3 – fish, soy beans, wheat germ, fortified milk, yogurt or eggs, beans, peas, tofu, nuts and seeds, canola oil, walnut oil and flaxseed oil

- lean protein – lean cuts of beef, lean ground beef, lean poultry (turkey, duck, chicken), lean pork and lean lamb

- antioxidants – black beans, pinto beans, berries, prunes, apples, pecans, sweet cherries, plums, cooked russet potatoes and artichokes

The trick is to keep everything balanced and avoid the foods that can worsen your fibromyalgial discomfort.

Foods to Avoid

Taking careful considerations on the foods to avoid can help a lot in alleviating the symptoms of fibromyalgia. Take note of the foods to eliminate in your diet and you will gain freedom from this debilitating condition.

Stop or minimize your consumption of sugar and artificial sweeteners. It's best to opt for stevia, a healthy and natural alternative for sugar without causing any trouble. You can also use natural sugar substitutes such as honey, agave syrup or even coconut sugar. Ultimately, sugar is a sweet poison to the body that causes inflammation and other diseases.

Drinks that contain caffeine must also go. Coffee, cola drinks and other caffeinated beverages should be avoided if you want to keep the pain away. If drinking coffee can't be avoided, choose the decaffeinated one. Keep in mind that caffeine can also be found in certain pain and cold medications so read their labels first before taking any of them.

Flavor enhancers like MSG and preservatives like sodium nitrate are bad news for people with fibromyalgia. To avoid foods that contain them, stay away from processed and canned foods and eat home-cooked meals instead when going to work or school.

It is also recommended to avoid milk-based products for a week if you have fibromyalgia. If you observe an improvement of your condition then you can do away with them. Get your daily dose of calcium from soy milk, tuna, broccoli, and salmon.

Eliminating gluten from the diet may also significantly improve the condition of some fibromyalgia patients. Anyone who would like to try a gluten-free diet should avoid pasta, grains, and white bread that contain wheat, barley or rye. These can be substituted with gluten-free alternatives such as corn or rice. Almond flour or coconut flour can also be used in baking instead of the usual wheat flour. Also, take note that some sauces may also contain gluten. Pay attention to ingredient labels. Wheat is surprisingly found in many products where you wouldn't think it would be.

Salt is also one thing that people with fibromyalgia should avoid. Experts know that bland food can make you lose interest in the whole endeavor therefore it is recommended to try eliminating salt in the diet gradually. Patients can also experiment with different salts, such as sea salt or Himalayan salt. Herbs and spices can also be used in creating unique flavors.

Monitor the foods that work best for you. It is best to keep a food journal and list down the foods that you have taken for the day and the events that happened on that particular day. Also, take special note of stress levels and the severity of the symptoms of your fibromyalgia.

Food Journal for Tracking Foods to Avoid

Creating a food journal is a great way to track your diet and changes in your symptom patterns. Include the following information in your food journal:

- Date

- Pain Scale (rate from 1 to 5 or 1 to 10)

- Details/Symptoms

- Food Eaten/# of Servings

- Triggers/Notes

Meal Guide

Sometimes it is difficult to plan for a healthy diet without a guide. The information below can help plan the right meal to take to ease the symptoms of fibromyalgia.

1. Fruit

Amount per Serving

-medium sized fresh fruit, one piece

-1/4 cup or 63 ml preserved or dried fruit

-1/2 cup (125 ml) fresh, frozen or canned fruit

Number of Servings

-ideally 4 or 5 per day

2. Greens

Amount per Serving

-1 cup raw green, leafy vegetables
-1/2 cup of cooked veggies, make sure not to overcook
-170 ml fruit or vegetable juice (preferably fresh)

Number of Servings
-ideally 4 or 5 per day

3. Grains

Amount per Serving
-a slice of bread (try spelt, buckwheat or corn bread)
-1 ounce dry cereal
-1/2 cup or 125 ml cooked cereal, pasta (try rice, corn or quinoa flour) or rice

Number of Servings
-ideally 6 to 8 per day

4. Fats

Amount per Serving

-1 tbsp (15ml) low-fat mayonnaise

-2 tbsp or 30 ml light salad dressing

-5 ml semi-melted margarine (that's about 1 tsp)

-1 tsp (5 ml) vegetable oil

Number of Servings
-ideally 2 to 3 per day

5. <u>Seeds, including nuts and legumes</u>

Amount per Serving

-1/3 cup (1.5 oz.) nuts (like almonds, pistachios, and peanuts)

-2 tbsp or 1/2 oz. sunflower seeds or other seeds

-1/2 cup cooked dry peas, beans or lentils

-2 tbsp or 30 ml peanut or almond butter

Number of Servings

-4 or 5 per week

6. <u>Lean meat, poultry, fish or seafood</u>

Amount per Serving

-1 ounce cooked lean meat, skinless poultry, fish or seafood

-1 egg

-1 ounce canned tuna in water without added salt

Number of Servings
-3 or less per day

Meal Plan

The meal plan below serves as your guide in planning your meal for the day (taken from the above meal guide).

Fruit (4-5 servings per day)

Breakfast: 170 ml fresh fruit juice

Snack (Optional): one fresh fruit

Lunch: ½ cup canned fruit

Snack (Optional): ¼ cup preserved fruit

Dinner: can add another serving here if desired

Greens (4-5 servings per day)

Breakfast: can have one serving here if desired

Snack (Optional): handful of cherry tomatoes

Lunch: 1/2 cup cooked mixed veggies

Snack (Optional): 170 ml fresh vegetable juice

Dinner: 1 cup raw green leafy vegetables

Grains (6-8 servings per day)

Breakfast: 3 slices of bread

Snack (Optional): 1 ounce dry cereal

Lunch: 1/2 cup steamed rice

Snack (Optional): 1 rice cake

Dinner: 1 cup cooked pasta

Fats (2-3 servings per day)

Breakfast: a tsp of semi-melted margarine

Dinner: olive oil salad dressing with a dash of lemon

Seeds including nuts and legumes (4-5 servings per week)

Breakfast: sprinkle flax seeds or chia seeds on your cereal or a smoothie; spread almond or peanut butter on your toast

Snack (Optional): almonds or pumpkin seeds

Snack (Optional): peanut butter or almond butter

Lean meat (2-3 servings per day)

Breakfast: 1 poached egg

Lunch: 2 ounces fish

Snack (Optional): 1 hard boiled or scrambled egg

Dinner: 2 ounces lean meat

Ways to Enjoy Your Meat

The best way to cook your lean meat is by grilling, steaming or broiling. Avoid frying them as much as possible and if you need to add some sugar or salt, keep it minimal.

For fish, it can be steamed and served with a light mayo dip to enjoy a succulent dish.

For added taste, you can also prepare a dry rub for the meat – a bit of salt, chili powder and pepper. Spread the dry rub all over the meat then grill or broil it. Prepare a light salad to complete your meal. The dry rub goes well with any meat including fish. Create some variations in taste by squeezing a lemon or lime on the meat before cooking.

As you go along with the planning and preparing of the healthy dishes to keep the symptoms of fibromyalgia under control, you will see that everything will become natural and easier to you.

Following a healthy meal plan will not only improve the symptoms of fibromyalgia but the overall fitness and health as well (not to mention the bonus of having a slim and fit body).

It is said that it takes 21 days to break a habit. Try maintaining your dietary changes for at least 21 days to see results. Expect to have symptoms of withdrawal if you choose to cut out caffeine, sugar, dairy or wheat. Sometimes you may feel worse before you actually feel better. Stick with it because it will soon pass and the reward will be worth it.

Chapter 9 - Recipes to Try

Gone are the days when eating healthy and nutritious food is synonymous with something bland and unappetizing. With some help from these great healthy recipes and good meal planning, putting an end to the hardships brought about by fibromyalgia will just take a fraction of time.

Here are some recipes to try and include in your meal plan. You can divide the prepared food to eat during lunch and dinner, just make sure not to go way beyond the suggested serving portions.

Berry Salad and Blackened Chicken

You will need:

2 ounces of skinless chicken breast

1/2 tsp mixture of blackening spice

½ head romaine lettuce

Vegetable toppings (radish, grated carrots, tomato, peas, pea pods, red cabbage and pepper strips)

fruit toppings (raspberries, blueberries and strawberry slices)

olive oil

vinegar or lemon dressing

Procedure:

Get the chicken breast and rub it with the blackening spice mixture. Grill until internal temperature has reached 165°F. Prepare the salad base using the romaine lettuce. Top with the vegetable toppings, then the fruit toppings. Add oil and vinegar dressing or olive oil with lemon dressing. This is good for a single serving.

Tuna Salad Platter

You will need:

1 ounce canned tuna in water

1/4 cup celery, chopped

2 tbsp light mayonnaise (or yogurt for a healthier choice)

1 hard boiled egg

bell pepper strips, shredded cabbage, cherry tomatoes, grated carrots

1 cup romaine lettuce, divided in two parts

Procedure:

Mix tuna, celery, mayonnaise and egg then set aside. Toss half of the romaine lettuce at the bottom of a salad bowl and top with half of the sliced vegetables. Toss in the other half of the romaine and then half of the sliced vegetables. Add in the previously prepared tuna and mayonnaise dressing.

Tuna Salad with Jalapeño

You will need:

1 6-ounce canned tuna in water, drained

1 tbsp light mayonnaise (or yogurt for a healthier choice)

1 small jalapeño, diced and without seeds

1 small tomato, diced

1/2 tbsp lime juice

1/4 onion, finely chopped

Procedure:

Put tuna in a bowl then add mayonnaise and onion. Mix them well. Add the remaining ingredients and serve.

Grilled Crunchy Chicken

You will need:

2 ounces chicken breast, with the skin on

A clove of garlic

Seasoning mix without salt

Aluminum foil

Procedure:

Rub the chicken breast with garlic and the salt-free seasoning. Heat the grill using medium heat. Make a "boat" for the breast using the aluminum foil. Put the chicken in the boat and place the aluminum boat on the grill. Cook for 45 minutes while turning the chicken inside the boat every fifteen minutes. When chicken turns golden brown, serve.

This makes 2 servings.

Stuffed Colorful Peppers

You will need:

3 pcs bell pepper (red, green, and yellow)

350 grams lean ground beef or sirloin

1 egg

2 tablespoons oat bran

1-2 cloves garlic, crushed

1 tsp paprika

Procedure:

Preheat your oven to 356°F or 180°C. While preheating your oven, cut your bell peppers in half, lengthwise. Deseed the bell peppers. Line your roasting tin with wax paper or greaseproof paper. Arrange your sliced bell peppers on the tin. Bake them for approximately 10-15 minutes. While baking your bell peppers, prepare the beef stuffing. In your food processor, place your beef, egg, oat bran, paprika and garlic. Mix these ingredients well. In the absence of a food processor, you may also mix the ingredients in a bowl. Use a fork to mix well. Take out the bell peppers from the oven and let them cool a bit. Stuff them with the beef mixture and put them back in the oven. Bake for approximately 20-30 minutes or until the beef mixture is done.

Mushroom Burger

You will need:

8 oz. of lean ground beef or sirloin

6-8 pcs Portobello mushroom

2 tablespoons oat bran

2 strips low fat bacon

1 tablespoon flaxseed

1 teaspoon olive oil

Procedure:

In a bowl, mix all ingredients well except the mushroom and bacon. Form patties out of the mixture. Grill your patties and bacon. Remove the stems of your mushrooms. Arrange your stemless mushrooms on a pan neatly. Set your stove on medium-high and cook your mushroom until the juices come out. Place one burger patty on two mushrooms. Add the bacon on top of the patty then top it with another mushroom.

Egg and Spinach Scramble

You will need:

1-2 eggs, beaten

½ cup baby spinach, chopped

¼ teaspoon cumin

1 small clove of garlic, minced

½ medium-sized white onion

½ tablespoon dried onion

1 teaspoon virgin coconut oil

Procedure:

Mix the eggs, baby spinach, cumin and dried onion in a bowl. In a heated pan, put your virgin coconut oil and sauté garlic and onion. Add the egg mixture. Cook for 2-3 minutes.

Primal Breakfast Burrito

You will need:

4 egg whites

1 to 2 tomatoes, finely chopped

½ medium-sized onion, finely chopped

1 red pepper, cut into strips

¼ cup canned and diced green chilies

½ a cup of cooked meat (you can use ground beef, sliced steak or shredded chicken)

¼ cup of chopped cilantro

hot sauce or salsa

1 avocado cut into wedges

Procedure:

First, whisk your egg whites. Then, lightly oil a 10-inch skillet and warm this over a low fire. Slowly pour half of your egg whites onto the pan, making sure to swirl it so that it gets spread evenly and thinly. Cook it for about a minute until it resembles a tortilla before removing it from the pan. This would be your burrito wrapper. Using the same pan, sauté your onions in oil before adding the red pepper, tomato, green chili and meat. Whisk more of the egg yolks into this and turn it into a scramble along with your other ingredients. Spoon half of this filling into your wrapper and roll it up nice and tight. Add some avocados on top and serve with salsa or hot sauce.

Veggies with Spinach Artichoke Dip

You will need:

10 ounces frozen and chopped spinach

2 14-ounce cans of artichoke hearts

half a red bell pepper

1 teaspoon garlic powder

1/2 cup cashew butter

1 tablespoon of green onion

¼ teaspoon cayenne

1 teaspoon salt

Procedure:

Cook your frozen spinach over medium heat, slowly breaking it up while it cooks. Add your red bell and artichokes and mix until everything is heated through. Then, add in your butter, cashew, garlic, cayenne, salt and green onion. Stir thoroughly and evenly. Serve this with your choice of veggies or veggie chips.

Sesame Seed Crusted Snapper

You will need:

6 to 7 ounces Red snapper, filleted and skinned

1 tablespoon sesame seeds

kosher or sea salt,

fresh black pepper (cracked)

1 tablespoon of grass-fed butter

Procedure:

Dust one side of the snapper fillet with a mixture of kosher salt and pepper before laying it on top of the sesame seeds. Press down to ensure an even coating. Do the same to the other side. In a frying pan, melt a teaspoon of the butter. Increase the heat before putting the snapper in the pan, cooking each side for at least 3 to 4 minutes. The seeds should take on a golden color.

Honey Orange Chicken

Ingredients:

1 pound chicken breast, cubed

2 tablespoons garlic

2 tablespoons ginger

2 tablespoons honey

2 tablespoons coconut aminos

1 tablespoon chili sauce

1/2 cup orange juice

green onions, chopped

fish sauce for seasoning

How to:

Stir fry your chicken in the coconut oil until it begins to brown. Add your garlic and ginger then sauté for 1 minute. Lower your heat and add the liquid ingredients. Stir everything to coat the chicken evenly and allow to simmer until the sauce thickens. Serve with green onions.

Spinach and Ham Omelet with Spicy Piperade

You will need:

coconut oil

2 eggs already beaten

salt and pepper

1 cup ham, cubed

at least a handful of baby spinach torn into small pieces

Procedure (Omelet):

Melt your coconut oil using a small sauté pan then add your eggs. Season the eggs with some salt and pepper. Cook it until your egg has set then sprinkle it with ham and pile on the spinach to one side. After you've placed the ham and spinach on one side, fold the egg. Top this with piperade.

You will need (Piperade):

3 cloves garlic

a large onion

3 tablespoons olive oil

4 sprigs of thyme

1 red bell pepper

1 yellow bell pepper

1 red chilli

1 cup cherry tomatoes

1 teaspoon salt

Procedure (Piperade):

Sauté your garlic, onions and thyme in the olive oil and wait until your onion begins to soften. After, add your chilli and peppers, continue to sauté this for at least 3 more minutes before finally adding the tomatoes. Sprinkle some salt to taste before covering and letting it simmer for at least 5 minutes.

Mango Avocado Spiced Chicken Salad

You will need:

1 small lettuce

1 to 2 cups of shredded chicken

1 diced avocado

1 diced mango

½ teaspoon cumin

½ teaspoon chili powder

salt and pepper for seasoning

Procedure:

Place your lettuce in a bowl and do the same to your chicken in a separate one. Add a tiny bit of water to your chicken to keep it moist before microwaving for at least 15 seconds. Add the chili and cumin to this and mix. Once done, add it to your lettuce and simply top with some avocadoes and mangoes. You can add a light dressing such as olive oil and lemon juice, or eat as is.

Conclusion

Thank you again for purchasing *"Fibromyalgia Book Guide."*

I hope this book was able to help you find treatments and strategies on how to successfully live with fibromyalgia and manage your pain.

The next step is to apply these strategies and make the necessary changes to your diet. It's shocking how the food we eat has such profound effects on the body -especially sugar. I'm amazed by how much better my body feels after cutting sugar out of my diet even for just 2 weeks. Although it was incredibly difficult for me to do, I came to a point of desperation which propelled me to make the changes necessary for my health.

Finally, if you want free books and want to know what some of my friends and I are up to, please like our Facebook page: www.facebook.com/joypublishing

Sincerely,

Mia Soleil

Mia   Soleil

Preview Of "Guide to Pain Management: How to Achieve Pain Relief and Live Pain Free for Life"

Pain and the Body

When you cut yourself, blood oozes out and there's a sharp pain that follows. If you have a migraine, you feel a chronic throbbing pain in your head. If you are burnt, pain is intensely unbearable. These are different scenarios where a person undergoes a painful experience. Pain in varying degrees of intensity and frequency is identified. The definition of pain, however, is out of the question.

What is pain?

Pain is a complex stimulus. There is no exact definition because it is an entirely subjective sensation. It is the foremost reason why people seek medical attention. Pain tells you that something is wrong or damaged. The International Association for the Study of Pain defines it as "an unpleasant sensory and emotional experience associated with actual or potential tissue damage or described in terms of such damage".

In actual context, pain is not always associated with physiological processes. Medical attention can identify and treat physical pain, but there's also another kind of pain which is really hard if not impossible to treat through medical means...emotional pain. So what is pain? Pain, to put it simply, is far more than neural transmission and sensory transduction. It is a complex mixture of emotion, sensation, culture, experience and spirit.

How does the body react to pain?

Pain perception or nociception is the process where a painful stimulus is signaled and relayed to the central nervous system from the point of origin. It is entirely different when compared to normal stimuli like touch, ordinary pressure and temperature. When the stimulus is non-painful, normal somatic receptors are the first to act. If it is a painful stimulation, nociceptors are the first to fire up.

This process includes several steps:

1. Point of origin or contact with stimulus- the point of origin can be mechanical such as cuts, pressures, abrasions and pressure. It can also be chemically inflicted like burns.

2. Reception – It is a process where the nerve ending senses the stimulus.

3. Transmission – When nerve endings sense the stimulus, they transmit the signal to the central nervous system through a series of neurons.

4. Perception – This is where the brain receives the signal for further processing and action.

When you cut your hand, there are several factors that contribute to your perception of pain. First is the mechanical stimulation of the sharp object that cut you. Your cells are damaged and they release potassium. This is why you feel the intense sharp pain at the moment of injury. Then Prostaglandins, histamines and bradykinins from the immune cells invade the area during inflammation. This is the stage where your body is protecting you from the foreign stimulus. You will experience a longer dull ache or numbing feeling along the affected area.

Nociceptor neurons travel in peripheral sensory nerves. The signals are relayed from the free nerve endings at the layer of the skin. These signals are sent to the spinal cord through the dorsal roots. They synapse on the neurons within the spinal cord segment and also two or three segments below and above the point of entry. This is basically the reason why it is sometimes difficult to locate the location of the pain in the body especially when the damage is internal.

Secondary neurons then transmit the signal upward through the spinothalamic tract. The signal travels from the spinothalamic tract to the medulla (brain's system) and ends in the thalamus, which is the central relaying center of the brain. Some neurons also send signal to the medulla's reticular receptors which control the physical behavior.

Once the signal is processed in the brain, some signals will pass through the motor cortex, to the spinal cord then down to the motor nerves. These impulses cause muscle contractions that make you move your hand away from the object.

What are the types of pain?

There are different types of pain. Neuroscientists and physicians classify pain in three ways:

1. Acute pain- This is a type of pain which is inflicted to the body. An injury to the body like a cut or burn causes an acute pain in the affected area. It warns of potential damage and compels action from the brain. It can develop slowly or quickly. Depending on the type of injury and the

intensity of the damage, pain can last up to a few minutes to a year. When the wound starts to heal however, acute pain goes away.

2. Chronic pain – It is a persistent kind of pain. It does not require your body to respond unlike acute pain. Chronic pain still persists even when the trauma has been healed. It lasts longer than six months. An example of a chronic pain is a migraine.

3. Cancer/malignant pain – This is a kind of pain associated with ...

Check out the rest of this book on Amazon.

Or go to: http://amzn.to/1eP7QRh

Check Out My Other Books

Below you'll find some of my other books that are popular on Amazon and Kindle as well. Simply click on the links below to check them out. Alternatively, you can visit my author page on Amazon to see other work done by me.

Eczema Treatment Guide: How to Live Pain Free with Natural Eczema Treatments and Eczema Diet Recipes

Pain Management Guide: How to Achieve Pain Relief and Live Pain Free for Life

One Last Thing...

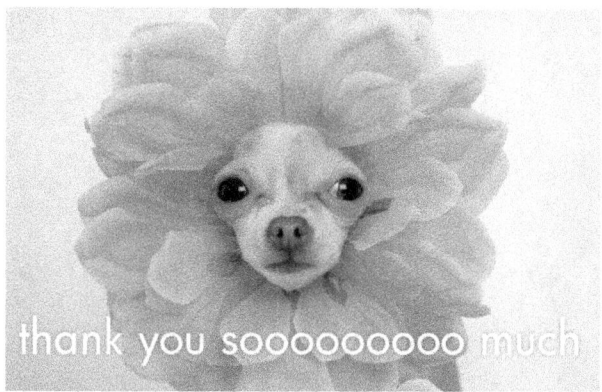

If you believe that this book is worth sharing, would you please take the time to let others know how it affected your life? If it turns out to make a difference in the lives of others, they will be forever grateful to you, as will I.

www.ingramcontent.com/pod-product-compliance
Lightning Source LLC
Chambersburg PA
CBHW070606290526
45790CB00002B/808